Distribution, publication, and copying in any form are prohibited and subject to damages.

TEN HYPNOSES

Copying, publishing, and sharing with third parties are only permitted with the written consent of the author. Please observe the notes on copyright and usage.

Distribution, publication, and copying in any form are prohibited and subject to damages.

Copying, publishing, and sharing with third parties are only permitted with the written consent of the author. Please observe the notes on copyright and usage.

Ingo Michael Simon

TEN HYPNOSES

44

Deep Relaxation

Distribution, publication, and copying in any form are prohibited and subject to damages.

© 2024 Ingo Michael Simon
All rights reserved.
Independently published
www.ingosimon.com

Important Notes for Urgent Attention:

The contents of this book are based on the practical experiences of the author with hypnosis applications and psychotherapy in a trance state. Although the author has strived for the utmost care, errors or misunderstandings in the presentation cannot be completely excluded. Therapeutic work with people and the application of hypnosis are solely the responsibility of the hypnotist. It cannot be ruled out that parts of this book may be misunderstood or that the application of a presented procedure may cause an undesirable reaction in the client. The author also assumes no co-responsibility if work with a client is carried out with reference to the statements in this book.

The Author:

Ingo Michael Simon studied psychology and education and is a hypnotherapist with practices in southwestern Germany and Switzerland. With the help of hypnosis-supported psychotherapy, he primarily treats people with persistent psychological conditions. His practice focuses on anxiety disorders, pathological compulsions, and psychosomatic illnesses. His therapeutic offerings mainly include classical and modern hypnosis applications and the dreamland therapy he developed himself.

Copying, publishing, and sharing with third parties are only permitted with the written consent of the author. Please observe the notes on copyright and usage.

Distribution, publication, and copying in any form are prohibited and subject to damages.

INTRODUCTION	**6**
COPYRIGHT AND USAGE	**8**
HYPNOSIS 1	**10**
HYPNOSIS 2	**15**
HYPNOSIS 3	**21**
HYPNOSIS 4	**26**
HYPNOSIS 5	**31**
HYPNOSIS 6	**36**
HYPNOSIS 7	**40**
HYPNOSIS 8	**45**
HYPNOSIS 9	**51**
HYPNOSIS 10	**56**
ALL TITLES IN THE SERIES	**62**

Copying, publishing, and sharing with third parties are only permitted with the written consent of the author. Please observe the notes on copyright and usage.

Distribution, publication, and copying in any form are prohibited and subject to damages.

Introduction

The series "Ten Hypnoses" is very well known in Germany, Austria, and Switzerland as a collection of texts for therapeutic work and is used by numerous psychotherapeutic practices, doctors, therapists, coaches, and other helping professionals. I am pleased to now be able to offer these texts in other countries as well.

Most therapists have their own methods for inducing and deepening trance as well as for exiting trance. Therefore, I have focused on the main part of the hypnosis. The texts in this book can be integrated as the main part into any hypnosis process. The texts in this collection use various hypnosis techniques. I will not explain these in detail, as I assume that users have the appropriate training. It is also not necessary to understand the exact structure or functioning of the different parts. The texts can simply be read aloud, and they will have their effect.

Decide for yourself which text best suits your client or patient at any given time. You can also combine passages from different texts. It is not about using all ten hypnoses in sequence. It is a selection of possibilities.

Copying, publishing, and sharing with third parties are only permitted with the written consent of the author. Please observe the notes on copyright and usage.

I want to emphasize that books cannot replace therapy. Psychotherapy or other therapeutic treatments involve much more. A careful diagnosis is the necessary basis for deciding on the use of methods, including whether hypnosis or one of my texts should be used. Even in this case, preparatory discussions, follow-up discussions during the session, and of course, a therapeutic concept for the sequence of sessions and the content approaches are essential parts of therapy. This cannot and should not be achieved with a collection of texts.

In any case, I wish you much success in your work and I am pleased if my text templates can contribute in a small way.

Ingo Michael Simon

Copyright and Usage

Copying, publishing, and sharing with third parties is prohibited and only permitted with the written consent of the author. Please observe the following copyright and usage guidelines.

This work has been carefully crafted and created to the best of the author's knowledge and personal experience. It comprises text templates and application guidelines for professional hypnosis sessions. The author is a licensed psychotherapist with extensive experience in psychotherapy, coaching, and personal training using hypnotic techniques and methods. Nevertheless, the author and the publisher assume no liability for the accuracy of information, instructions, and advice, nor for any typographical errors. The author and publisher accept no responsibility or liability for the application of these texts and recommendations with clients or patients, nor for any potential consequences or unexpected reactions. It is expressly noted that the application of therapeutic and advisory techniques and formulations lies solely and entirely within the responsibility of the practitioner. This also applies to adherence to the boundaries of legally regulated medical and therapeutic practices. The fact that a book containing action proposals is freely available for sale does not imply that its application with clients or patients is permitted for everyone.

Hypnosis 1

… … There is a special kind of relaxation … … a pleasant path that leads you into a very deep and cozy relaxation … … and along the way, you can truly unwind … … You can hear my voice clearly the whole time … … But maybe soon it won't matter what I say, and you'll simply sink into your feelings … … Yet, a part of you always listens attentively … … because actually, you can do both … … listen attentively and rest deeply … … so deeply that it might feel like a restful sleep … … with complete and truly lasting relaxation … … And after your deep relaxation, you'll feel fresh and energized … … as if you've had a refreshing vacation … …

… … Your subconscious supports you in your relaxation and recovery … … because your subconscious, just like your conscious mind, wants to experience true rest … … Now, you can bring to mind a very pleasant memory … … Remember a beautiful day in your life … … or choose a wonderful fantasy … … a dream that you love … … and imagine this pleasant memory, this lovely fantasy, now moving to the left side of your body … … and you follow these beautiful thoughts and memories to the left ... ... You follow these lovely and pleasant feelings to the left side ... ... Everything is beautiful on the left side ... ... And while you dream on the left side, in your beautiful images and fantasies, your subconscious moves into your right side ... ... all the way to the right ... ... You may now dream and deeply relax ... ... You may sleep if you want, on the left side are all the beautiful feelings and thoughts ... ... and your subconscious helps you rest deeply on the right ... ... Maybe your head moves a little to the left ... ... Let it happen ... ... Your head follows the pleasant feeling to the left ... ... And while all your thoughts and feelings dream only on the left side and become sleepier, your subconscious on the right side helps you rest and recover ... ... Go deeper and deeper into the beautiful state of calm ... ... into the completely safe state of inner peace ... ... and allow your deep inner self, your subconscious, to help you relax even more deeply ... ... Your subconscious can do this ... ... If you wish, let my voice fade into the background ... ... Everything is alright ... ...

... ... Now, you may enjoy the peace and simply dream in your beautiful inner images ... ... While you dream a beautiful and restful dream on the left side, your subconscious ensures optimal recovery on the right side … … Your subconscious hears words on the right side that optimally support your recovery … … while you dream on the left side … … The more you succeed in truly imagining beautiful and pleasant memories or fantasies on the left side and staying there, the more your subconscious ensures optimal recovery … …

… … Now, you can easily let go of all the burdens of everyday life … … Every exhale is now a release of tension and burdens … … With each breath, you let go of the stress of daily life and become freer … … and inner freedom is what allows you to relax deeply … … deeper and deeper … … Your deep inner self now lets you truly relax … … Everyday life fades into the distance … … Everyday life is already far away and disappears more and more … … While you rest deeper on the left side and sink deeper into pleasant feelings, your subconscious ensures the best recovery on the right side … … for new strength that will be available to you after awakening … … But now, you may rest … … relax deeper and deeper … … Deep peace is quite easy to achieve, and you achieve it now … … deep, deep peace … … On the left are all the beautiful images and feelings, on the right is wonderful recovery … … Dream on the left and recover on the right … … {Approx. 20-30 seconds of silence} … … And now, continue to enjoy the beautiful peace … … Peace and recovery are closely connected … … Every moment of deep peace leads to wonderful recovery … … and to new freshness for the day … … Enjoy the deep peace because it gives you freedom and recovery … … Isn't it wonderful how easy this is? … … Deep relaxation and recovery are that simple … … {Approx. 20-30 seconds of silence} … …

… … You've now experienced something very special, and your inner self has learned something truly beneficial for you … … You are in wonderful thoughts and feelings, and you are recovering … … because your subconscious is doing this for you … … And now, you can spread out your thoughts and all your images throughout your body again … … and your subconscious also spreads out throughout your entire body … … Thoughts, feelings, and subconscious flow gently into each other and become one … … Thoughts, feelings, and subconscious are one with you, and you are relaxed and already well-rested … … And from now on, inner peace and quick recovery with renewed strength are closely connected

… … So, every moment of rest leads to recovery and to new strength for the day … … Enjoy the peace … … until my voice brings you out of the trance and back to your waking day … … {Approx. 20-30 seconds of silence} … …

Hypnosis 2

+++ Guidelines for Implementation +++

The following hypnosis text is structured so that it can be used as a "regular" hypnosis session or as a self-hypnosis training. If you want to simultaneously teach your client how to perform effective self-hypnosis at home with this session, also read the sections {Only for self-hypnosis training}, which you can otherwise omit and still have a good hypnosis session for your practice. A self-hypnosis trigger is a signal that initiates the trance state. With its help, even an unpracticed client can continue working with self-hypnosis at home. Of course, they can work "only" with simple suggestions that they can easily remember and that we should prepare, or with simple visualizations. Triggered self-hypnosis is a very good tool to give the client something to work on between sessions and to support therapy. Thus, the time between sessions in practice is not without therapy but is continued at home. A completely self-directed self-hypnosis, without a trigger, is also learnable, but it requires a lot of time and practice. Setting up the trigger is a fairly simple task and certainly relieves the client, whom I don't want to burden with training a self-directed self-hypnosis. Despite all the naysayers, I also claim here that it's really no problem to teach a client simple trigger self-hypnosis. It's no more dangerous than meditation or autogenic training or yoga. People survive those at home unscathed as well. I've seen numerous patients in my practice who not only managed well with self-hypnosis but enjoyed it. And if a patient enjoys doing self-hypnosis, however simple the suggestion in the main part may seem, then that's very good support for compliance.

+++ End of Guidelines +++

… … … Today, your body can learn to relax very deeply … … … You will experience truly deep relaxation in just a few moments, and in fact, it has already begun … … But in just a few moments, your relaxation will go even deeper … … and your deep inner self, your subconscious, will learn how simple and quick very … … very deep relaxation can be … … This way, you will also be able to quickly enter a state of true relaxation and deep rest without hypnosis whenever you take a break and rest ... ... {Only for self-hypnosis training: ... You can even learn to do this hypnosis on your own, because that too is easy ...} ...

... ... You will easily enter a deeper relaxation ... ... Imagine a white rose against a black background ... ... a white rose against a black background ... ... Look at this rose ... ... Focus only on the white rose, as this will cause all thoughts to fade, and you will come to rest ... ... It's very simple ... ... Imagine the white rose against a black background and wait for the deep relaxation to set in ... ... Focus only on the white rose, and you will feel the deep relaxation ... ... Perhaps you already feel how the image of the rose is leading you into deep relaxation ... ... or you'll feel it more clearly in just a few moments ... ... {Only for self-hypnosis training: ... Whenever you close your eyes to find deep rest and then imagine the white rose against the black background, your body immediately enters a pleasant and comfortable trance ... just like now ...} ...

... ... You want to relax very deeply today ... ... Deep relaxation is especially restorative and can be like a truly restful vacation ... ... It leads you into a pleasant silence, almost like sleep ... ... and perhaps it even feels as if you're deeply asleep and only hearing my voice from afar ... ... That's completely fine because a part of you always listens to me and would follow my words attentively even in the deepest sleep ... ... Imagine yourself walking down a staircase, and with each step, you become sleepier, and with each step, your body relaxes even more ... ... and more ... ... and with each step, you say ... ... I relax once more deeply ... ... I relax twice more deeply ... ... I relax three times more deeply ... ... I relax four times more deeply ... ... I relax five times more deeply ... ... I relax six times more deeply ... ... I relax seven times more deeply ... ... I relax eight times more deeply ... ... I relax nine times more deeply ... ... I relax ten times more deeply ... ... and then you are in a very, very deep state of inner calm ... ... Now ... ... {Only for self-hypnosis training: ... This is how you deepen your trance at home, by walking down an inner staircase and counting just as you heard ...} ...

... ... You are already in deep peace, but if you want, this relaxation can go even deeper ... ... if you allow it, and if you truly want it, you will now relax very, very deeply ... ... Imagine finding such a deep inner peace that it feels like complete inner tranquility ... ... And with each breath, this inner peace spreads … … And then imagine saying with conviction … … … Today, I simply find inner peace … … Today, I find double inner peace … … Today, I find triple inner peace … … Today, I find fourfold inner peace … … Today, I find fivefold inner peace … … Today, I find sixfold inner peace … … Today, I find sevenfold inner peace … … Today, I find eightfold inner peace … … Today, I find ninefold inner peace … … Today, I find tenfold inner peace … … … And then everything feels very relaxed and calm … … very calm and very peaceful … … deeply relaxed … … {Only for self-hypnosis training: … And when you bring yourself into trance and deepen it, you can whisper this suggestion to yourself … just as you heard here today, whispering ten times … … I find inner peace today and counting … … simply … … doubly … … and so on until you say … … I find tenfold inner peace today … … That's how simple it is, and you can do it yourself …} … Now enjoy this state of deep calm and true relaxation … … Enjoy this wonderful state of inner peace that now fills you … … This is how it should be now … … Peace and tranquility … … deep peace and complete tranquility within you … … You have earned this peace … … You may now enjoy this peace, and you may return to this state of true relaxation anytime … … just as now … … exactly as now … … Approx. 20 seconds of silence …

{Only for self-hypnosis training} … … When you want to do self-hypnosis at home, you proceed exactly as you experienced here … … It is completely safe … … Start with the image of the white rose and imagine it until you feel that you are coming to rest … … Then whisper the suggestion to yourself … … I relax once, twice, and so on until you say: I relax ten times … … Then you go even deeper by whispering ten times: Today, I find inner peace … … Then you may rest, and to wake up, imagine yourself lying in the snow wearing a T-shirt and shorts, and then just say: I will wake up now – One – Two – Three … … Then you can open your eyes and be awake … … It's really that simple … … You will succeed just like here today … … You go into trance and wake up again quite easily … …

Hypnosis 3

… … With this hypnosis, you want to … deeply relax and experience truly good recovery … … … that's why you're so open to this nice and calm hypnosis … …

… … With this hypnosis, you want to … deeply relax and experience truly good recovery … … … that's why you also willingly sink into inner peace … …

… … With this hypnosis, you want to … deeply relax and experience truly good recovery … … … that's why you're already joyfully anticipating this deep calm … …

… … With this hypnosis, you want to … deeply relax and experience truly good recovery … … … that's why you gladly accept all relaxation suggestions … …

… … Your thoughts drift away like clouds in the sky, and … you just let them go … … … and that's why you get tired so quickly and want to sleep … …

… … Your thoughts drift away like clouds in the sky, and … you just let them go … … … and that's why you also feel the pleasant pull of the trance … …

… … Your thoughts drift away like clouds in the sky, and … you just let them go … … … and that's why you are now ready to sink deeply into yourself … …

… … Your thoughts drift away like clouds in the sky, and … you just let them go … … … and that's why it gets quieter and stiller within you … …

… … Now, you relax very deeply … … as in a deep, deep sleep … …

… … Your body has the need to relax even more deeply … … and that's why all your muscles release and you find deep peace … …

… … Your body has the need to relax even more deeply … … and that's why your tendons now relax, and you sink even deeper into relaxation … …

… … Your body has the need to relax even more deeply … … and that's why your joints now rest and feel the deep calm that fills you … …

... ... Your body has the need to relax even more deeply ... ... and that's why you now relax really deeply ... ... deeper than deep ... ...

... ... Now, you relax very deeply ... ... as in a deep, deep sleep ... ...

... ... Inner peace and deep, peaceful relaxation are the most pleasant feelings of this moment ... ... and that's why it's worth letting go more and more and dreaming ... ...

... ... Inner peace and deep, peaceful relaxation are the most pleasant feelings of this moment ... ... and these feelings you may now fully enjoy ... ...

... ... Inner peace and deep, peaceful relaxation are the most pleasant feelings of this moment ... ... and that's why this moment is also your moment of peace ... ...

... ... Inner peace and deep, peaceful relaxation are the most pleasant feelings of this moment ... ... and that's why you relax even more deeply ... ...

... ... Now, you relax very deeply ... ... as in a deep, deep sleep ... ...

… … You can now and every day experience peace … by taking time for yourself and finding inner calm … … … You just do it exactly as you are now … …

… … You can now and every day experience peace … by taking time for yourself and finding inner calm … … … You close your eyes, and relaxation happens … …

… … You can now and every day experience peace … by taking time for yourself and finding inner calm … … … You can experience every day what you are experiencing now … …

… … You can now and every day experience peace … by taking time for yourself and finding inner calm … … … You can relax deeply every day, just like now …

… … Now, you relax very deeply … … as in a deep, deep sleep … …

… … You have now found deep peace and relaxation, and with that, you recover and find new strength … … and from now on, every conscious moment of rest fulfills this purpose … …

… … You have now found deep peace and relaxation, and with that, you recover and find new strength … … and you clearly feel this strength when you are awake again … …

… … You have now found deep peace and relaxation, and with that, you recover and find new strength … … and from now on, every moment of rest will bring you real and noticeable recovery and real and clearly noticeable new strength … …

… … Now enjoy the peace and the recovery … … Enjoy your new strength … …

Hypnosis 4

… … This hypnosis is for deep relaxation … … your deep relaxation … … because now you need rest more than anything and want to recover … … The state of trance is very well suited for experiencing truly deep relaxation … … because first the body relaxes and comes to rest … … You can feel that clearly … … You feel the relaxation of your body, which has become so calm and loose … … and with every further breath, you let go even more, allowing yourself to glide into a very, very deep relaxation … … During this time, you can hear everything that is happening around you … … My voice guides and accompanies you … … and you understand every word I say clearly … … And all the words that help you achieve a truly very deep relaxation work immediately and help you relax even more deeply than you expected … …

… … You experience the deepest relaxation and peace best when you remember situations in which you have already found rest and relaxation … … Let's start with the situation right now … … Imagine it once more … … like in a dream … … like in a beautiful dream that you are dreaming right now … … in a deep sleep … … in deep inner peace … … You have laid down to relax … … Then you made yourself comfortable, laying down in such a way that you are really comfortable … … Maybe you moved around for a while, changing your position because you really wanted to relax deeply … … because you wanted to do everything in a way that would help you succeed in relaxing really deeply … … Over time, you came to rest, and your body became still … … Your body found a position like in a good sleep … … maybe lying on your back or on your side … … covered with a blanket … … and if you want, you can snuggle even deeper into your blanket … … or adjust a comfortable pillow under your head until it is just right … … That's how you did it, and it helped you come to rest … … Then you heard the induction of the trance, and the words of the trance induction helped you find a nice calm … … Every word helped you relax … … Every word relaxes you even now … … every word … … Then you heard the deepening … … During this, you went deeper and deeper into inner relaxation … … you felt how the words you heard gently and kindly guided you deeper … … and you let go … … let go as well as you could already, and perhaps even felt that in just a few moments, an even deeper relaxation and calm would set in ... ... That's how you relaxed ... ... That's how you relax again now ... ... and this time, you relax even more deeply ... ... This time, you go very, very deep into inner peace ... ... deeper than ever before, and you hear all my words clearly ... ... and you are here in complete safety ... ... You are doing well because you find wonderful peace ... ... You are doing well because you sink into a very deep inner relaxation and peace ... ... deeper and deeper ... ... and it is restorative ... ... You regenerate and recover wonderfully in this moment ... ... You have found your inner peace ... ... This is good ... ... This is really good ... ... {Approx. 20 seconds of silence} ... ...

... ... And now you remember a very relaxing day in your life ... ... a truly relaxing day it was ... ... maybe on a vacation ... ... or on a very special day that comes to mind spontaneously ... ... But you can take your time and just feel what you feel ... ... You don't need to have a visual memory now because your whole body remembers that one very special day of relaxation ... ... and you feel the feeling of relaxation and recovery in your body ... ... because every memory leads to our body remembering and feeling the feeling of the remembered time ... ... and your body now feels the relaxation and recovery ... ... You feel the relaxation and recovery now ... ... Now everything is calm within you ... ...

... ... You now feel deep within yourself and perceive your feelings clearly ... ... feelings of peace ... ... feelings of recovery ... ... of regeneration ... ... The whole weight of the day now falls away from you, and you feel free ... ... You feel your breath flowing clearly, you perceive every breath clearly ... ... the inhalation ... ... and the exhalation ... ... and every exhalation frees you because now you can truly exhale every disturbing thought ... ... Breathe out and feel liberated ... ... That's right ... ... You are doing it right ... ... This is how you find truly good and restorative peace ... ... All thoughts flow away with your breath, and you become free ... ... Every single breath frees you ... ... frees you completely ... ... You feel free and feel new strength ... ... You feel completely free and feel new, fresh strength ... ...

... ... With this feeling of regeneration and fresh strength after this deep relaxation, you now focus on your bodily sensations ... ... You feel your body in the here and now ... ... Everything is completely alright ... ... You rest within yourself

… … and soon you can face your everyday life again with new strength and new energy … … Feel the peace of your body … … Feel the freedom within you … … Feel the regeneration and the new strength … …

Hypnosis 5

… … You have the desire to relax very deeply now, to find truly restorative peace and discover new strength in the depths for the challenges of daily life … … You have the desire for deep relaxation … … and with that, you also have the intention to relax very deeply … … It is your will … … It is your goal to relax deeply … … now, to relax very deeply … … And for this, you don't need to do anything … … Just let my words take effect … … Let the words you hear simply flow into your inner self and let them unfold their positive and constructive effect for your well-being … … Listen to the words that help you with deep and calm relaxation … … and above all … … Don't help me with this … … Let yourself be helped to relax … … How easy and simple it is for you now … … and this ease, this relief, you have truly earned … … because now nothing else is important … … Everything now happens for your well-being, and everything serves only your recovery … … Now is time just for you … … Now is really time just for you … …

… … You have often experienced that it's not so easy to relax deeply … … But with a suitable image, everyone can relax well … … So, you can relax with the right image too … … The right image for your relaxation is a tree with a thousand leaves on it … … an autumn tree with a thousand brown and yellow leaves that will soon be shed and fall to the ground … … And everything that can burden you in your thoughts is like the leaves on this tree … … So, imagine each of the thousand leaves as a little burden in your thoughts … … You know the disturbing thoughts and worries that often occupy you so that you cannot always relax deeply with ease … … … Over time, so many heavy thoughts have accumulated that you couldn't always fully process … … They hang like wilted, long unnecessary leaves on the tree of your thoughts, and each withered leaf is a disturbing thought … … … It's time to let these leaves go … … and with them, let all disturbing thoughts fall into the depths … … and with the falling leaves, let all worries disappear into the depths … … They may fall away from you … … and tumble to the ground like leaves falling from a tree in the autumn wind … … So, imagine the tree … … Imagine it with a thousand leaves that you can free the tree from … … in your imagination … … and as you imagine it this way, letting go of disturbing thoughts succeeds, and you sink deeper and deeper into the depths of the trance … … Your breath is the wind that loosens the leaves from the tree and gently guides them into the depths … …

… … Now, imagine the tree with the leaves as clearly as you can … … Look at it before your inner eye … … The more you succeed in imagining a tree with a thousand leaves, the deeper you can relax now … … Your breath blows like an autumn wind around this tree … … Every exhale becomes the wind that loosens the leaves from the tree … … with every breath, more leaves loosen from the tree and tumble into the depths … … … Now, all the leaves and all the thoughts you immediately recognize as disturbing thoughts are loosening … … They loosen as withered leaves from the tree and slowly tumble in the autumn wind into the depths … … Many leaves sink slowly to the ground, carried by the autumn wind … … and the deeper these leaves sink, the closer they get to the ground, the deeper you relax … … the deeper you sink into the calm and restorative trance … … Some leaves turn slowly as they fall … … tumbling dreamily and playfully in the wind, and then gently falling into the depths ... ... and with them, you also sink into very deep relaxation ... ... Then, leaves and thoughts loosen that you cannot quite grasp, but your deep inner self knows which thoughts as disturbing thoughts are now to be ended ... ... Hundreds of withered leaves gently loosen with the next breath and tumble into the depths ... ... and you sink deeper and deeper with them ... ... Some leaves turn slowly as they fall ... ... tumbling dreamily and playfully in the wind, and then gently falling into the depths ... ... and with them, you also sink into very deep relaxation ... ... deeper and deeper ... ...

... ... Finally, all the leaves loosen from the tree in the autumn wind ... ... The tree sheds all its leaves ... ... Your inner tree of thoughts now sheds all thoughts and hands them over to the autumn wind that gently guides them into the depths ... ... A thousand leaves tumble in the wind to the ground ... ... They turn and bounce in the wind, finding a gentle and calm path into the depths ... ... You watch the leaves and observe their path into the depths ... ... and you yourself sink deeper and deeper into a beautiful state of inner peace ... ... With every breath, it becomes quieter within you ... ... With every leaf that sinks to the ground ... ...

gently and safely carried by the autumn wind, you also sink deeper ... ... gently and safely carried by my voice ... ... and by your deep inner self ... ... A thousand leaves slowly float to the ground ... ... and each individual leaf draws you into peace and relaxation with it ... ... With each leaf that reaches the ground, you become calmer ... ... and sleepier ... ... very sleepy ... ... as sleepy as in a deep sleep ... ... in a deep and very restorative sleep ... ...

... ... This deep relaxation gives you wonderful and restorative peace ... ... and deep within you, you find new strength for life's challenges ... ... But just focus on feeling the peace ... ... Everything else happens by itself ... ... because you know ... ... In peace lies strength ... ... Deep within peace lies strength ... ... and you truly feel peace now ... ... You feel a truly pleasant and deep peace ... ... There lies the strength for the waking day ... ... There, in the peace, lies the strength for all challenges ... ... So, enjoy the beautiful and deep peace ... ... Enjoy the new strength ... ...

Hypnosis 6

… … … You want to relax deeply today … … because deep inner peace is what you need most right now … … and deep inner peace is good for you … … … Now, you attune all your senses to peace … … You listen within and let all the noises outside become quieter … … Only my voice is still important … … because my voice guides you into deep peace … … Now, it's all about your relaxation … … your deep, deep relaxation … … With each breath, you relax more deeply … … and with each breath, you feel the inner peace more clearly and enjoy this beautiful state … …

… … Surely you know that we are most successful in what we can truly imagine … … and besides, we succeed fastest in what we can believe in the most … … It is our beliefs and convictions that lead us to our goals … … Your goal is to be able to relax deeply today and whenever you want … … And it is easy for you to believe that you can relax deeply because you have often rested and found deep relaxation in your life … … You have experienced deep peace and relaxation before … … You experience deep peace, for example, whenever you fall asleep, because real relaxation happens in sleep ... ... What it's about now is achieving such relaxation in trance ... ... It's about achieving a state of rest that goes as deep as a deep sleep ... ... only faster ... ... and without actually sleeping ... ... For this, you can use an affirmation ... ... a belief statement that acts like a ritual for you ... ... Affirmation means reinforcement ... ... or confirmation ... ... You can use a confirmation formula to repeatedly find a pleasant peace ... ... even more peaceful than now ... ... Now you already feel tired and relaxed, and you have the desire to simply rest ... ...

... ... Now, pay attention to your body sensation ... ... Turn your attention with full awareness and mindfulness to your feeling ... ... and prepare for your peace affirmation ... ... because while your inner peace deepens, your deep inner self is waiting to hear your peace affirmation and make it your own ... ... That's exactly what happens when you can accept it and want to accept it ... ... when it is good for you and helps you relax and reach deep peace ... ... And that's exactly what it's there for ... ... to achieve truly deep peace ... ... That is your goal ... ... that's why you are listening to this hypnosis ... ... to really relax deeply ... ... You hear the affirmation, and you repeat it internally ... ... {{5-10 seconds pause}} ...

... ... I open myself to the silence within me and allow myself to gently fall into the depth of the trance – Now ... ...

Now, take a deep breath ... ... and exhale slowly and long ... ... once more ... ... {Now, in the client's breathing rhythm} ... ... deep inhale ... ... and slow, long exhale ... ... This allows the valuable affirmation to penetrate deeper ... ... This way, the words of relaxation you heard can become more your own ... ... This way, this attitude can become deep truth within you, and you can actually experience this feeling of deep peace and feel it ... ... you can feel the deep peace within you now ... ... deep peace that is now possible ... ... deep peace that is now very easy ... ... deep peace that is now especially comfortable ... ... So, this new connection is formed within you ... ... This way, your affirmation becomes your confirmation of will and your declaration of intent ... ... and your inner truth ... ... the truth of deep and truly restorative relaxation ... ... Deep relaxation ... ... That is your path and your experience today ... ... Deep relaxation for you ... ...

… … Deep within your inner center, in the place of silence and peace, these helping words are at work, which have become your attitude of trust and peace … … You hear and confirm them once more in the depth … …

… … I open myself to the silence within me and allow myself to gently fall into the depth of the trance – Now … …

… … Now, take a deep breath in and out … … Let your breath flow calmly and enjoy the deep peace … … enjoy only the deep peace … … deep, deep peace … …

… … So good … … It is time … … Your whole body has attuned itself to the effect of your belief, to the effect of the affirmation, which you confirm with your inner attitude and your will … … And your peace affirmation now helps you, and again and again, to relax deeply and immediately … … especially and even when you think it might not be so easy to achieve deep relaxation, it leads you into the depths and carries you there safely, and you experience wonderful recovery … …

Hypnosis 7

… … You want to experience deep relaxation … … deeper and faster than you usually know … … and above all, you want to let go of disturbing thoughts to really be able to enjoy the relaxation and peace … … because deep and restorative relaxation is only possible when your thoughts recede more and more into the background … … That's why you chose hypnosis … … because you are convinced that this way you can enter a deeper form of peace and regenerate much faster and more sustainably … … You can experience two forms of peace, and only both together lead to truly restorative peace … … the physical relaxation that has already begun with the induction and deepens with each word you hear … … and the mental relaxation, the letting go of thoughts, and this too has already begun with the hearing of the introductory words of this trance … … and this mental peace also goes deeper and deeper with every word you hear … … Now you can go the way into very deep relaxation by focusing more and more on the feeling and perception of your body … … on the already existing peace of your body, because a calm body also makes all thoughts calmer and leads you into deep relaxation ... ...

... ... Now pay attention to your body, feel along your body and feel the peace and relaxation of your body ... ... Feel also the peace and relaxation of your body ... ... Feel how your body feels now because there is already the feeling of deep peace within it ... ... When we come to rest, become very tired, and sleepier, our body becomes sluggish and slow ... ... our body shows us that it wants and can relax even more deeply ... ... Your body shows you this feeling now ... ... Perceive it ... ... Now perceive your body feeling of peace ... ... Feel your body parts and check which part has already found the most peace ... ... Feel your head and check how calm it has already become ... ... very calm perhaps ... ... Then feel your shoulders and check how they feel ... ... how much peace can already be felt in your shoulders ... ... But maybe there is a body part or a spot that is even calmer and already much more relaxed ... ... maybe your arms ... ... or the legs ... ... or your abdomen is deeply peaceful ... ... Feel your body, and you will find the area that now feels the most relaxed ... ... You find a spot in your body that feels the most peaceful ... ... Here you feel the physical relaxation best

... ... Here lies also your potential for peace, wherever that may be ... ... and if you are not quite sure, choose the body part that you spontaneously and most closely associate with peace ... ... And focus entirely on this spot, entirely on this area because there is peace ... ... Send all your mindfulness and attention there because that is your peace center ... ...

... ... You have found the peace center of your body ... ... or you have simply determined it ... ... That works too, because body and thoughts are closely connected ... ... So, focus on this area of your body and feel the peace there ... ... Let the relaxation and peace you feel there in your body now become even more clear in your consciousness ... ... Let the peace and relaxation you feel there in your body now become the peace of your entire organism ... ... Feel how the deep inner peace spreads ... ... like a pleasant warmth that spreads from this spot in your body and envelops your whole body ... ... This way, your entire body becomes just as tired and just as calm as this one spot that became tired first ... ... like this one spot that was the first to perceive the relaxation ... ... Peace spreads throughout your entire body ... ... Your inner zone of peace becomes bigger and bigger ... ... Your inner zone of peace spreads out ... ... Your comfort zone becomes bigger and bigger ... ... and the feeling of deep, deep relaxation takes up more and more space ... ... You feel the inner peace more and more clearly ... ...

... ... You become calmer and enjoy a truly deep relaxation ... ... a truly deep relaxation of your body ... ... a truly deep relaxation of your thoughts ... ... a truly deep relaxation of your feelings ... ... That's good ... ... Let your peace find its way ... ... deeper and deeper peace ... ... deeper and deeper peace ... ... That's a good feeling ... ... That's your relaxation ... ... That's your peace ... ... That's your inner stillness ... ... That's your recovery ... ...

Now, enjoy the peace and relaxation ... ... Enjoy the relaxation of your body and your thoughts ... ... and trust that from now on you can always enjoy the relaxation and peace of your body just as quickly and even faster ... ... just as in deep sleep ... ... Trust that from now on, you can also always enjoy the relaxation and peace of your thoughts just as quickly and even faster ... ... just as in sleep ... ... just as in deep sleep ... ...

... ... And whenever you lay down to relax deeply and want to recover as quickly as possible, your body will remember to relax and find deep peace just as today ... ... just as quickly and even faster than today ... ...

Hypnosis 8

+++ Guidelines for Implementation +++

An anchor {or trigger} is a stimulus that is meant to create a specific feeling or evoke a particular thought. It is a signal that is perceived by the client and then triggers an internal process. The established anchor then replaces the suggestion. In everyday life, a client can use an anchor to trigger or create a desired state, even without a trance state. Numerous stimuli can be used as anchors/triggers. I work with the following possibilities, which I also use in the "Ten Hypnoses" series:

Body anchors {Closing the hand, pressing the ball of the thumb ...} Visual anchors {Symbols, word cards ...} Acoustic anchors {Signal sounds like mobile phone ringing, melodies ...} Olfactory anchors {Essential oils ...} Haptic anchors {Hand smoothers, talismans ...}

I also distinguish between peri-hypnotic and post-hypnotic anchors. Peri-hypnotic anchors are those that are primarily used during hypnosis, with the therapist setting the anchor and then repeatedly triggering it as a complement to the suggestions and visualizations. Post-hypnotic anchors are mainly set up for use after the session so that the client can help themselves with them.

+++ End of Guidelines +++

… … You have a goal … … You have a clear intention for this hypnosis … … … You want to relax … … You want to relax very deeply … … deeper than usual … … … and that is possible today … … For this, I will show you a very special approach … … I will show you a trance anchor … … A trance anchor is a tool with which you can experience much deeper relaxation and peace today than you might have thought … … a very simple tool … … and this very special trance anchor is a tool that you can use at any time again … … also and especially outside of trance when you just want to truly rest … … because the trance anchor works like a switch that brings your body into a very deep and truly pleasant state of inner peace … … So, it is that today you learn how to activate your inner peace with the really simple and highly effective trance anchor … … You activate your new peace program with the anchor, and the anchor is just as easy to use as pressing a light switch to turn off the light ... ... This switch is located in your body ... ... and you trigger it with your hands ... ... You just need to know when and where to place your hands to trigger a quick and deep relaxation ... ... You will learn that now ... ...

... ... Now you feel calm and relaxed ... ... That's good ... ... very, very good ... ... because that's how it must be if you want to find and experience truly deep peace ... ... That's how it must be if you want to relax more deeply than ever before ... ... It must be this calm and remain so ... ... Now feel the peace and let it become very clear ... ... Perceive the inner peace that you already feel ... ... and if you think it should become even calmer within you, just take a deep breath in and slowly and long exhale ... ... because then it becomes automatically calmer ... ... all by itself, calmer ... ... Now my voice helps you ... ... because now you only need to follow my voice with some trust and with the desire for even deeper relaxation ... ... This way, you can now experience truly beautiful, deep peace ... ... This way, you can now experience a very pleasant state of inner peace and inner freedom ... ... But you can relax even more deeply with your anchor … … and you can relax even more deeply at any time … … You can always use your anchor, even and especially without trance, because once you have set it up with me, guided by my voice, it works securely and reliably … … and helps you always and everywhere to experience truly restorative relaxation if you so wish … … just like now, because now you also want to experience restorative relaxation … …

… … Now, in true relaxation and peace, everything around you becomes unimportant … … Now, it's all about this feeling of peace and your anchor … … Now, place your left hand on your solar plexus, so that your thumb rests on your breastbone and your index and middle fingers can feel your ribs … … This way, your palm rests on the solar plexus, the solar plexus of the body … … And now your body responds to the warmth radiating from your hand … … Feel the warmth radiating from your own hand and touching your body there … … and feel the peace and relaxation within you … … Let the feeling of peace become clear … … Perceive it consciously … … Now, as soon as you place your right hand on your left hand and apply a gentle pressure, as if you wanted to press a switch, you immediately go deeper into the relaxation you already feel … … Now, place your right hand on your left hand … … Feel the inner peace and deepen it by gently pressing your right hand onto your left hand … … … This way, you relax more deeply … … this way, you relax more deeply now … … deeper and deeper … … You find an ever deeper and wonderful inner peace … … and your subconscious mind stores exactly this effect of your anchor … … This is your deep relaxation anchor … …

… … Now, once again, put your hands to your sides and lay them next to your body … … because now you can use your anchor in complete calm to relax even more deeply … … To do this, take a deep breath in and slowly and long exhale and feel how deeply you have already relaxed … … Once again … … deep inhale and slowly and long exhale … … Good … … And now place your hands once more on your body … … first the left hand and over it the right … … And then press gently a few times with your right hand on your left and feel this gentle pressure in your solar plexus because that leads you deeper and deeper into the trance … … {Please wait until the client performs the movements} … … Feel how the gentle pressure of your own hand leads you into a very deep trance … … and enjoy this deep trance, this wonderful relaxation ... ... And if you think you have already reached a truly pleasant state of peace and you just want to enjoy the peace and sleepiness you feel, then just let your hands rest on your body and enjoy the peace ... ... Enjoy the peace ... ... Your deep inner self, your subconscious, has firmly set up the anchor for you ... ... You can use it at any time for yourself, even and especially without trance ... ... just as here and today ... ... just as here and today ... ... Your anchor works ... ...

Hypnosis 9

… … You want to reach a truly deep and very restorative trance today … … and in fact, you are already on your way there … … To experience a truly pleasant and very deep relaxation today, you have chosen hypnosis … … So, you have also dealt with hypnosis and realized … … Hypnosis is a special path … …

… … Experienced meditation teachers know it even better … … They know … … Suggestions heard in trance unfold helpful effects … … and you can use support and help for very deep relaxation … … because that's your goal, your intention … … You seek deep relaxation … … want to switch off and rest … …

… … And if the experienced meditation teachers are right, then the next step is inevitable … … You find this deep relaxation … … That's the next step … … A big step into the depths and peace … … That's the next step … …

… … Many people wonder what a trance feels like exactly and how one can notice being in a trance … … If you were sure that you were already in a truly deep trance, you would probably think ... ... You can feel the trance ... ... and you can also feel that it goes deeper ... ...

... ... In the state of trance, you can establish a special connection with your subconscious and use this connection for yourself ... ... for your quick and very deep relaxation ... ... You can communicate your wishes to your subconscious ... ... and once the special connection between your subconscious and you is established, it will fulfill your wishes ... ... Feel your body sensation and notice how it feels ... ... Maybe you already feel quite a pleasant relaxation ... ... If you can feel relaxation and you've been relaxing for a few minutes now, then you also feel ... ... the special connection to your subconscious is already there ... ... or you'll feel it in a few moments ... ...

... ... So, if you want to relax very, very deeply now, you can communicate the wish to your subconscious, for example ... ... that all disturbing thoughts should fall away from you ... ... You can even go further, because if ... ... the special connection to your subconscious works ... ... you can also wish ... ... that all thoughts should now fall away from you ... ... and once you can feel that it becomes quiet within, you can also recognize … … Now the way is clear for deep relaxation … …

… … If you imagine relaxation as a path you could walk into your deep inner self, you would always have a very simple path to deep relaxation … … Imagine you want to relax deeply, just like now, and … … You just take the direct path into the depth … … You can simply go directly into the depth … … Just imagine it … …

… … And once you have successfully walked this path, you know exactly … … Deep relaxation is very easy to achieve … … and … … You can relax very, very deeply … … … Sometimes it wasn't so easy to really come to rest, but today you have already managed to become calmer … … … today you really succeed … in experiencing a beautiful trance that is completely calm and restorative … … … Today it works for sure … something … to experience peace … … either … … as deeply relaxed … as you want or even … more deeply relaxed than ever before … who knows … …

… … Relaxation is a very personal matter, and everyone has their own access to it … … If you feel during this hypnosis that you have reached a point of good and restorative relaxation for yourself, you can clearly recognize ... ... This hypnosis has really led you into a special form of relaxation because ... You are experiencing deep relaxation in your feelings, in your emotions ... ...

... ... The words you hear now work very deeply, and their effect unfolds more and more ... ... Once their effect is fully unfolded, you feel ... ... You are very deeply relaxed, and you feel good ... ...

... ... In deep relaxation, you feel very calm and serene on the one hand, and on the other hand, there is an additional special feeling ... ... You feel very comfortable ... in deep trance ... It is a feeling of protected peace ... ... It is a feeling of security ... that you can feel in a deep trance ... ...

... ... If you now listen deeply into yourself and pay attention to your feeling, then maybe you can already say ... ... You feel this deep peace ... and ... You feel the restorative relaxation ... ... But even if you wouldn't quite feel it that way yet, you can trust the trance because ... ... With every breath, the relaxation goes deeper ... once it has begun ... ...

... ... You have surely already recognized ... ... Hypnosis is a good way to find inner peace ... ... this can be quickly achieved ... ... There is always a personal and individual way ... ... You find your good way ... ... in your own feeling ... ... Deepest relaxation is possible this way ... ...

Hypnosis 10

… … You want to experience a very pleasant and restorative relaxation now … … Maybe you want to relax so deeply that all thoughts fall away from you, and you don't think about anything at all because … … that's how recovery is best possible … … For this, you have chosen the path of hypnosis … … Good hypnosis helps you with good suggestions … … with words and phrases that gently and securely guide you into deep relaxation because … … in deep relaxation, you find the best recovery … … Words that sound familiar work the fastest … … These are the most effective suggestions … …

… Hypnosis is a … special path … {5-10 sec. pause} …

… Suggestions unfold … helpful effects … {5-10 sec. pause} …

… You find this deep … relaxation … {5-10 sec. pause} …

… You can feel the … trance … {5-10 sec. pause} …

... And you can also feel that it goes ... deeper ... {20-30 sec. pause} ...

... Hypnosis is a ... special path ... {5-10 sec. pause} ...

... Suggestions unfold ... helpful effects ... {5-10 sec. pause} ...

... You find this deep ... relaxation ... {5-10 sec. pause} ...

... You can feel the ... trance ... {5-10 sec. pause} ...

... And you can also feel that it goes ... deeper ... {20-30 sec. pause} ...

... You can communicate your wishes to your ... subconscious ... {5-10 sec. pause} ...

... The connection to your ... subconscious ... is established ... {5-10 sec. pause} ...

... All disturbing ... thoughts ... should fall away from you ... {5-10 sec. pause} ...

... The connection to your subconscious ... works ... {5-10 sec. pause} ...

... ... All ... thoughts should ... now fall away from you ... ... {5-10 sec. pause} ...

... ... Now the way is clear for the ... deep relaxation ... ... {20-30 sec. pause} ...

... You can communicate your wishes to your ... subconscious ... {5-10 sec. pause} ...

... The connection to your ... subconscious ... is established ... {5-10 sec. pause} ...

... All disturbing ... thoughts ... should fall away from you ... {5-10 sec. pause} ...

... The connection to your subconscious ... works ... {5-10 sec. pause} ...

... All ... thoughts should ... now fall away from you ... {5-10 sec. pause} ...

... Now the way is clear for the ... deep relaxation ... {20-30 sec. pause} ...

... You just take the direct path ... into the depth ... {5-10 sec. pause} ...

... You can relax very, very ... deeply ... {5-10 sec. pause}

...

... Today ... you really succeed ... {5-10 sec. pause} ...

... Today it works ... for sure ... {5-10 sec. pause} ...

... ... so ... deeply ... relaxed ... deeper ... than ever before ... ... {5-10 sec. pause} ...

... ... This hypnosis has led you ... into relaxation ... ... {5-10 sec. pause} ...

... ... You are experiencing deep relaxation ... in your emotions ... {20-30 sec. pause} ...

... You just take the direct path ... into the depth ... {5-10 seconds pause} ...

... You can relax very, very ... deeply ... {5-10 seconds pause} ...

... Today ... you really succeed ... {5-10 seconds pause} ...

... Today it works ... for sure ... {5-10 seconds pause} ...

... so ... deeply ... relaxed ... deeper ... relaxed than ever before ... {5-10 seconds pause} ...

... This hypnosis has led you ... into relaxation ... {5-10 seconds pause} ...

... You are experiencing deep relaxation ... in your emotions ... 20-30 seconds pause ...

… You are … very deeply relaxed, and you feel good … {5-10 sec. pause} …

… You feel … very good … {5-10 seconds pause} …

… It is a feeling of … protected … peace … {5-10 sec. pause} …

… It is a feeling of … security … {5-10 sec. pause} …

… … With every breath, the relaxation goes deeper … … {5-10 sec. pause} …

… … So, deepest relaxation is … possible … {20-30 sec. pause} …

… You are … very deeply relaxed, and you feel good … {5-10 sec. pause} …

… You feel … very good … {5-10 seconds pause} …

… It is a feeling of … protected … peace … {5-10 sec. pause} …

… It is a feeling of … security … {5-10 sec. pause} …

… … With every breath, the relaxation goes deeper … … {5-10 sec. pause} …

... ... So, deepest relaxation is ... possible ... {20-30 sec. pause} ...

Distribution, publication, and copying in any form are prohibited and subject to damages.

All Titles in the Series

Volume 1: Smoking Cessation
Volume 2: Anxiety and Restlessness
Volume 3: Burnout
Volume 4: Reducing Overweight
Volume 5: Coping with the Past
Volume 6: Suicidal Thoughts and Attempts
Volume 7: Psycho-Oncology
Volume 8: Obsessions and Tics
Volume 9: Self-Confidence and Decision-Making
Volume 10: Grief Work
Volume 11: Psychosomatics
Volume 12: Chronic Pain
Volume 13: Depressive Thoughts
Volume 14: Panic Attacks
Volume 15: Domestic Violence, Victim Support
Volume 16: Post-Traumatic Stress
Volume 17: Exam Anxiety and Stage Fright
Volume 18: Anti-Violence Training, Offender Support
Volume 19: Addiction Tendencies
Volume 20: Social Phobia and Fear of Contact
Volume 21: Nail Biting
Volume 22: Self-Awareness and Self-Love
Volume 23: Teeth Grinding and Night Clenching
Volume 24: Feelings of Guilt
Volume 25: Fear in Crowds
Volume 26: Fear of Flying, Aviophobia
Volume 27: Fear in Enclosed Spaces, Claustrophobia
Volume 28: Tinnitus, Ear Noises
Volume 29: Fear of Heights
Volume 30: Neurodermatitis

Copying, publishing, and sharing with third parties are only permitted with the written consent of the author. Please observe the notes on copyright and usage.

Volume 31: Finding Inner Balance
Volume 32: Overcoming Loneliness
Volume 33: Fear of Illness, Hypochondria
Volume 34: Anticipatory Anxiety, Fear of Fear
Volume 35: Jealousy in Relationships
Volume 36: Driving Anxiety
Volume 37: New Start after Separation
Volume 38: Fear of Injections
Volume 39: Heart Anxiety Neurosis
Volume 40: Overcoming Resentment and Anger
Volume 41: Resolving Blockages and Positive Thinking
Volume 42: Stress Reduction, Stress Management
Volume 43: Body Relaxation
Volume 44: Deep Relaxation
Volume 45: Fear of the Dark
Volume 46: Falling Asleep and Staying Asleep
Volume 47: Compulsive Buying
Volume 48: Restless Legs Syndrome
Volume 49: Bulimia
Volume 50: Anorexia
Volume 51: Overcoming Nightmares
Volume 52: Imagined Deformity
Volume 53: Overcoming Distrust, Finding Trust
Volume 54: Processing Failures
Volume 55: Humiliation, Emotional Hurt
Volume 56: Distressing Compassion, Vicarious Suffering
Volume 57: Self-Forgiveness
Volume 58: Self-Awareness, Self-Confidence
Volume 59: Saying No
Volume 60: Assertiveness
Volume 61: Setting Boundaries and Self-Assertion
Volume 62: Decision-Making Ability

Volume 63: Success Orientation
Volume 64: Ruminating, Circular Thinking
Volume 65: Accepting Pregnancy
Volume 66: Birth Preparation
Volume 67: Spiritual Opening
Volume 68: Joy of Life and Inner Lightness
Volume 69: Patience and Inner Peace
Volume 70: Fibromyalgia and Rheumatism
Volume 71: Irritable Bowel Syndrome, Crohn's Disease
Volume 72: Fear of Nausea, Emetophobia
Volume 73: Stuttering and Cluttering, Speech Flow Disorders
Volume 74: Concentration and Knowledge Anchoring
Volume 75: Vitality and Spontaneity
Volume 76: Searching for Meaning and Finding Goals
Volume 77: Life Crises, Life Events
Volume 78: Workaholism, Goal Obsession
Volume 79: Helper Syndrome, Helpless Helpers
Volume 80: Medication Abuse
Volume 81: Gambling Addiction
Volume 82: Internet Addiction, Smartphone Addiction
Volume 83: Hoarding Disorder, Compulsive Collecting
Volume 84: Conspiracy Thoughts, Overvalued Ideas
Volume 85: Fear of Operations and Treatments
Volume 86: Fear of Aging
Volume 87: Travel Anxiety
Volume 88: Anxiety When Urinating, Paruresis
Volume 89: Fear of Intimacy and Togetherness
Volume 90: Fear of Blushing
Volume 91: Coming Out in Homosexuality
Volume 92: Charisma Training
Volume 93: Migraines and Chronic Headaches
Volume 94: Overcoming Allergies, Bronchial Asthma

Volume 95: Normalizing Blood Pressure
Volume 96: Compulsive Perfectionism
Volume 97: Sports Hypnosis, Motivation
Volume 98: Sports Hypnosis, Performance Enhancement
Volume 99: Determination and Focus
Volume 100: Encountering the Inner Child
Volume 101: Cravings, Binge Eating
Volume 102: Stimulating Metabolism
Volume 103: Bipolar Mood Swings
Volume 104: Borderline, Identity Crises
Volume 105: Hypomania, Euphoria, Mania
Volume 106: Restlessness, Agitation
Volume 107: Nervous Breakdown
Volume 108: Adjustment Disorders
Volume 109: Self-Alienation, Depersonalization
Volume 110: Ending Self-Pity
Volume 111: Primary Gain of Illness
Volume 112: Secondary Gain of Illness
Volume 113: Bullying, Victim Support
Volume 114: Letting Go of Envy and Jealousy
Volume 115: Fear of Spiders, Arachnophobia
Volume 116: Fear of Dogs or Cats
Volume 117: Fear of Strangers, Xenophobia
Volume 118: Excessive Worries, Generalized Anxiety
Volume 119: Strengthening Sense of Responsibility
Volume 120: Unrequited Love, Heartache
Volume 121: Work-Life Balance
Volume 122: Letting Go of Unattainable Goals
Volume 123: Allowing and Accepting Help
Volume 124: Letting Go of Adult Children
Volume 125: Tourette Syndrome
Volume 126: Life Changes and New Starts

Volume 127: Accepting Life in a Wheelchair
Volume 128: Understanding and Overcoming Homesickness
Volume 129: Understanding and Overcoming Wanderlust
Volume 130: Dizziness, Meniere's Disease
Volume 131: Overcoming Aggression
Volume 132: Cutting and Self-Harm
Volume 133: Hair Pulling, Trichotillomania
Volume 134: Postpartum Depression
Volume 135: For Relatives of Dementia Patients
Volume 136: Self-Harm, Artificial Disorders
Volume 137: Activating Self-Healing Powers
Volume 138: Preventing Depression Relapse
Volume 139: Reactive Psychoses, Follow-Up
Volume 140: Obsessive Thoughts and Impulses
Volume 141: Compulsive Checking
Volume 142: Compulsive Counting, Symmetry Obsession
Volume 143: Compulsive Washing, Cleanliness Obsession
Volume 144: Compulsive Questioning
Volume 145: Dissociative Paralysis
Volume 146: Phantom Pain
Volume 147: Overcoming Complaining
Volume 148: Hay Fever, Pollen Allergy
Volume 149: Sexual Abuse, Victim Support
Volume 150: Standing Strong Against Sexism, #metoo
Volume 151: Binge Eating
Volume 152: Overcoming Thoughts of Revenge
Volume 153: Detachment from the Aggressor, Stockholm Syndrome
Volume 154: Courage to Separate
Volume 155: Chronic Fatigue, Exhaustion
Volume 156: Fear of the Future, Existential Anxiety
Volume 157: Excessive Worry About Children
Volume 158: Fear of Failure

Volume 159: Ending Distrust and Control
Volume 160: Dejection, Dysphoria
Volume 161: Boreout, Chronic Boredom
Volume 162: Bipolar Disorders, Relapse Prevention
Volume 163: Mania, Relapse Prevention
Volume 164: Nihilism, Feelings of Worthlessness
Volume 165: Thumb Sucking
Volume 166: Being Brave
Volume 167: Being Proud
Volume 168: Overcoming Shyness
Volume 169: Being Able to Delegate Responsibility
Volume 170: Being Able to Show Emotions
Volume 171: Letting Go of Guilt, Victim Support
Volume 172: Processing Guilt, Offender Support
Volume 173: Mood Swings, Cyclothymia
Volume 174: Lack of Drive, Vital Sadness
Volume 175: Hearing Voices with Reality Reference
Volume 176: Confident Communication
Volume 177: Standing Up for Oneself
Volume 178: Taking New Paths
Volume 179: Confident Job Application
Volume 180: No Longer Being Taken Advantage Of
Volume 181: End of Submissiveness
Volume 182: Depressive Numbness
Volume 183: Mood Drops, Affective Incontinence
Volume 184: Mood Instability
Volume 185: Somatoform Disorders
Volume 186: Stomach Ulcer, Psychosomatic
Volume 187: Accepting Amputation
Volume 188: Overcoming and Letting Go of Hatred
Volume 189: Ending Accusations
Volume 190: Allowing Tears, Being Able to Cry

Volume 191: Finding and Sorting Repressed Feelings
Volume 192: Somatoform Pain
Volume 193: Living Autonomously
Volume 194: Anhedonia, Joylessness
Volume 195: Persistent Sadness
Volume 196: Obesity, Food Addiction
Volume 197: Parents of Abused Children
Volume 198: Letting Go and Letting Be
Volume 199: Childhood Sexual Abuse
Volume 200: Fear of Loss

www.ingramcontent.com/pod-product-compliance
Lightning Source LLC
Chambersburg PA
CBHW030501220526
45464CB00006B/2607